SIRTFOOD DIET
Cookbook

Eva Parker

Contents

Introduction

Before starting to read what, will become the definitive recipe for you, I would like you to pause for a moment to ask yourself a couple of questions: how many times have you felt uncomfortable with your body? How many times have you promised yourself that you would have changed your eating habits when you looked at yourself in the mirror or when you put on your bathing suit?

And after making this decision, how many times have you embarked on diets on the edge of the inhuman, which have massacred both your body and your psyche and your morale?

If your answer to these questions is "more than once" or "many times," rest assured, I understand the mistrust that you may feel towards diets. I went there too.

I also underwent rigorous diets over and over again, and I got. As a result, only losing time, happiness, and sometimes even health, only to lose a few pounds, and then take them all back (sometimes even more) once the diet is finished or stopped.

So, rest assured, I know that feeling of defeat too.

But it is precisely for this reason that I present this recipe book to you today. To share with you the fantastic revelation that I incurred when I came across this new diet, or rather this new lifestyle, which is the Sirt food diet.

I want to be honest with you, the first time I came across this new diet, coming from various negative experiences with other foods, I thought this had nothing different from the others, and it was nothing but just a way of setting a new trend. Fortunately, thanks also to my curiosity, I decided to try to understand more deeply why celebrities such as Adele and Pippa Middleton were so enthusiastic about it.

And after deepening my knowledge of the Sirt diet, through in-depth research on scientific texts and articles that explained the role comprehensively that "Sirtuins." I understood that my first impression could not be further from the truth.

Let me explain it better: on the market and the net, we now have access to a great deal of information, and a topic like that of weight loss and having a dream body, attracts much attention and is therefore much exploited, sometimes unfortunately also by charlatans without direct experience or adequate scientific training. It is consequently ubiquitous to come across a myriad of diets and the like, which have been put together quickly and not only, having no scientific assumptions, they prove ineffective, but they can also be harmful to our body, sometimes even so much. The real problem, with these diets, is that even if you can lose weight (and with what sacrifices), as soon as you stop the food, it takes only a few days to find yourself back to the starting point and sometimes even worse than as we were initially.

Because, let's be honest and let's face it, to lose weight, it is enough not to eat! And it is precisely on this strategy that most of the diets that have been in vogue in recent years are based.

So much so that most of the diets you can find around are mainly based on a meager daily calorie count, sometimes enhancing the dubious properties of some miraculous foods. And here I say suspicious features because the properties that are attributed to many of the so-called "super-foods" do not have any type of scientific foundation or research behind them.

In my opinion, and my experience, the goal of taking a diet should not only be to lose weight but to be able to build a new balanced and healthy way of eating and living.

And it is precisely for these reasons that the Sirt diet was created and developed, which is instead based on robust and proven scientific foundations. This new

8

diet, this modern philosophy, I dare say, allows us to have a broader approach to achieve the objectives mentioned above, that is to lose weight and improve our health. In a nutshell, to find our balance.

And this is precisely the journey that awaits us in this: understanding how the iteration of these proteins called Sirtuins, when we take them through certain foods that contain them in large quantities, manage to interact with our body and to activate what which is called the "skinny gene," to make us lose weight by only losing fat, and not muscle mass. Indeed, I assure you that by following the advice that you will find in this, your muscle mass will tend to grow, while you will lose fat.

And if this already seems a lot to you, it's not over yet. In this, you will also find more than one hundred recipes that will allow you to combine Sirt foods (i.e., those foods containing Sirtuins) to create delicious recipes that will satisfy your palate. And all this while you lose weight!

And what's more, all the foods recommended in this dietary program, are all fresh, whole grains, readily available and suitable for our palate which combined or with other ingredients give rise to tasty dishes.

To lose weight so quickly and effortlessly has never been more comfortable, more pleasant and healthier!

Phase 1

Hello to the Sirtfood Diet, Step 1. It's time for hyper success when you take massive action to create a leaner, leaner body. Follow our simple step-by-step instructions and use the delicious recipes you find. In addition to our regular 7-day program, we also have a meatless version that is suitable for vegetarians and vegans. Feel free to go with anything you want.

You will benefit from all the advantages of our clinically proven strategy of losing 7 pounds in phase 1 in seven days. However, note that this requires additional strength. So, don't just stick to the percentages on the scale. You also shouldn't get used to measuring yourself every day. In fact, in the last days of Phase 1, we often see dandruff increasing due to muscle growth, although the size continues to shrink. Therefore, we want you to look at the graphics but not control them. Find out how you feel in the mirror, if your clothes are snug, or if you need to tie a knot at the waist. These are all perfect measures of the underlying changes in your body composition.

Also consider other improvements such as well-being, energy level and smoothness of the skin. You can even have your cardiovascular and metabolic well-being tested at a local pharmacy to see improvements in factors such as blood pressure, blood sugar and lipids such as cholesterol and triglycerides. Aside from losing weight, incorporating sort foods into your diet is a big step towards making your cells healthier and more susceptible to disease, and preparing for an extraordinarily balanced life.

How to Follow Phase 1

We will guide you through the seven-day program every day to make Phase 1 as simple as possible, including information on green sort food juice and delicious recipes that are easy to follow every step of the way.

This phase of the Sirtfood diet includes two different aspects:

Days 1 to 3 are the most important, and you can eat up to 1000 calories per day during this period, including:

- Sirtfood juice three times green
- The main course

On days 4 to 7, your daily food intake increases to a maximum of 1,500 calories, consisting of:

- Sirtfood twice green juice
- Two main dishes

There are very few laws to follow the diet. For continual progress, the main thing is to integrate it into your lifestyle and your daily life. But here are some simple but useful tips for the best result:

1. Take a good juicer

The juice is an essential aspect of the diet, and a juicer is one of the best health cares purchases you can make. While price should be the deciding factor, some juicers can extract juice more efficiently from green leafy greens and herbs, with the Breville brand among the best juicers we've tested.

1. Start the preparation

One thing stands out from the multitude of comments received: those who planned were the best. Learn more about products and techniques and buy the essentials. You will be amazed at how natural the whole cycle is with everything that is planned and ready.

2. Save your valuable time.

If time is short, dress well. Meals can be prepared the evening before. Juices can be made in bulk and stored in the refrigerator for up to three days (or longer in the freezer) until the content of sirtuin-activating nutrients begins to decrease. Just protect it from light and add it when you can eat it at the party.

3. Eat early

Eating early in the day is healthier, and hopefully, food and drink should not be consumed after 7 p.m. However, the plan is mainly based on lifestyle, and late eaters still enjoy great benefits.

4. Place the juices

These should be taken at least an hour before or two hours after a meal to maximize the digestion of green juices and distribute them throughout the day instead of being close together.

5. Eat until you are satisfied.

Sips can have a dramatic impact on appetite, and some people will be satisfied before their meals are finished. Listen to your body and feed until you are full instead of cutting all the calories. Because Okinawa has been around for a long time, he says, "Feed before 80 per cent is done."

6. Take advantage of the diet.

Don't get stuck on the end goal, but stay on track. This lifestyle consists of enjoying food in all its splendor, for its health benefits, but also the pleasure and pleasure that it offers. Research shows that we are much more likely to be successful if we focus on the path rather than the ultimate goal.

Beverages

In addition to the recommended daily serving of green drinks, another phase 1 drinks may be easy to drink. Calorie-free drinks, usually regular juice, black coffee and green tea. If your usual taste is black or herbal teas, you can also add them. Fruit juices and soft drinks remain. Alternatively, try adding a few sliced strawberries to sparkling or still water to prepare your strong, healthy drink if you want to spice things up. Keep it in the fridge for a few hours, and you will have a surprisingly refreshing selection of sodas and juices.

One thing to keep in mind is that we are not suggesting abrupt and significant changes in your daily coffee consumption. Caffeine withdrawal symptoms can make you feel bad for a few days. Likewise, significant increases can be painful for those who are particularly sensitive to the results of caffeine. They also recommend drinking coffee without adding milk, as some researchers have found that adding milk reduces the absorption of beneficial nutrients that activate sirtuin. The same has been observed with green tea, but the incorporation of lemon juice increases the absorption of its nutrients activating sirtuin.

Keep in mind that this is the most auspicious time and that you should feel calm when you know that it only takes a week; you should be a little more careful. We have alcohol for this week in the form of red wine, but only as a heating element.

Sirtfoods Green Juices

Green juice is an integral part of the phase 1 sirt diet program. All the ingredients are healthy sirt foods, and each juice gives you a powerful blend of natural compounds like apigenin, kaempferol, luteolin, quercetin and EGCG which work together to activate your sirtuin genes and promote loss of fat. We have added lemon to it, as its natural acidity has been shown to prevent, stabilize and improve the absorption of nutrients that activate Sirtuin. We also add a touch of apple and ginger to taste. But both are available. However, some people find that once they get used to the taste of the fruit, they altogether remove the apple.

Sirtfood Green Juices (1 serving)

- Two handfuls of kale (about two and a half ounces)

- A handful of arugulas (one ounce or 30 g)

- A small handful of parsley leaves (about 5 g)

- Two to three large celery stalks (five and a half ounces or 150 g), including the leaves

- Half a medium green apple

- Piece of fresh ginger 1 to 2.5 cm

- Half a lemon juice

- Half a teaspoon of matcha powder *

- Days 1 to 3 of phase 1: only added to the first two juices of the day

- Days 4 to 7 of step 1: added to both juices

Remember, although we weigh all quantities exactly as described in our pilot test, in our experience, a handful of measurements work exceptionally well. In fact, they are best suited for adjusting the number of nutrients to a person's body size. Larger people tend to have more massive legs and therefore receive a proportionately higher volume of dietary nutrients to meet their body size, and vice versa for smaller people.

- Collect the vegetables (kale, arugula and parsley) and mix them. We think juicers can vary in efficiency when compressing leafy greens and you may need to rejuvenate the leftovers before switching to the other ingredients. The goal is to get about 2 ounces of material or about 1/4 cup (50 mL) of green juice.

- Now mix the celery, apple and ginger.

- You have to cut the lemon and also pass it through the juicer, but it is much easier for us to put the lemon in the juice by hand. At this point, you should have a total of about 1 cup (250 ml) of juice, maybe something else.

- Only when you have extracted the juice and are ready to serve, add the theme. Pour a small amount of juice into a bowl, then add the matcha and mix vigorously with a fork or whisk. In the first two drinks of the day, we only use matcha because it contains small amounts of caffeine (the same quality as a normal cup of tea). If it's wasted late, you can keep it awake with those who aren't used to it.

- Once the matcha has dissolved, add the remaining juice. Give it a final mix, and the juice is ready to drink. Easy to fill with running water as desired.

On days 1 to 3, you can take the juices at different times of the day, then have a standard meal at the time that suits you best (preferably lunch or dinner).

Here is the 1-7 Day Phase 1 Meal Plan.

Phase 2

The four-week program is already starting to have some positive effects on your body weight. If you managed to pass the first week of this program (allow me to congratulate you), the remaining phase would be a walk in the park for you. This phase is less radical than the seven-day meal plan, and you have the chance to increase your calorie intake by adding a third meal slightly so that you can get used to it in the long run. This phase should last between two and three weeks, so it is up to you what you want from it. If you are not satisfied with your weight loss, then you can repeat the seven-day meal plan in the last week of this program. If you are happy with the results, you can just extend phase 2 for the fourth week as well.

This stage of the program will allow you to lose weight more sustainably. You can have three meals per day, increase your calorie intake (still, I wouldn't go higher than 2,000 to 2,500 calories per day), and have just one green juice per day. This is where you have more liberty to choose the meals from your meal diet, will include the meals included per day so that you can reap most of the benefits of this diet.

Since you are having three meals per day, let's start with scheduling your meals. I would recommend having breakfast between 7:00 and 7:30 a.m. Lunch should be served in the afternoon and 1:00 p.m., and dinner between 6:00 and 7:00 p.m. I would recommend having the green juice around 3:00 p.m. You should have dark chocolate (85 percent cocoa) as dessert, but you can also go with a few strawberries and walnuts. Don't forget to drink two cups of coffee per day (depending on the size of the container, you can double the amount), but don't forget about matcha green tea or water with strawberries. Since you have to keep the calorie intake very low (between 2,000 and 2,500 calories), consuming lots of salads is required. You simply can't go wrong with a salad, especially when it is rich in sirtuin-activating nutrients. Don't forget to add some extra-virgin olive oil to make the mixture even more powerful.

I will include a detailed meal plan for this phase (breakfast, lunch, and dinner), but if you are not satisfied with the weight loss, or you simply love green juices, and you want to have more, you can simply go ahead and follow phase 1 in the fourth week of this plan. This is your call, and as you can see, step 2 is a bit more flexible than stage 1. The meal plan for phase 2 can be used as guidelines, so it is not mandatory to respect it as you would obey the law. If you prefer a specific sirtfood meal, then you can insert it into your meal plan. It also includes some ideas on snacks, juices, smoothies, cakes, desserts, salads, dressings, and soups.

However, let's reveal some of the details of the maintenance phase. This is the period when you will consolidate the results of your weight loss, but the weight-loss process doesn't end with the first week. You will continue to burn fat in this phase of the program. One of the most striking things about this diet is that the fat you lose will be compensated by muscle gain. So yes, you will look a lot leaner, old clothes will fit you again, and you will receive plenty of compliments from people who know you. But keep in mind that the health and weight loss benefits can continue long after the four-week program if you choose to stick to this diet.

Typically, phase 2 should last two weeks, but if you enjoy it that much, you can stick to this phase, or you can simply use the first-week meal plan in week 4. During this phase, you are laying the foundation of your lifelong health. Maintenance is an essential part of this program, as it helps your body adjust to the sirtuin-activating way. This phase should include three main meals, one or two sirtfood snacks, and one green juice. The diet principles still apply, so you need to eat early. Avoid any calorie intake by 7:00 p.m. After this hour, you can only have noncaloric drinks like water or green tea. Sleep is essential with any meal plan, so I wouldn't recommend having coffee after 7:00 p.m.

Although counting calories is more related to the first week of the program and the founders of this diet don't encourage the calorie count, I wouldn't exaggerate with the meals too much. Indeed, you are allowed to have three meals per day, but you still need to be careful with the quantity. When it comes to drinks, there is a whole variety you can try, but remember to stay away from sodas and fruit juices, mostly because of their high concentration of sugar and other chemicals. If you want to drink fluids, you will need to stick to the sirt green juices. Don't forget about matcha green tea, black coffee (preferably with no sugar, milk, or cream added), and water. If you have the chance to drink a glass of red wine at dinner, don't miss this opportunity, as that glass comes with plenty of benefits. Remember to stick to one glass; do not drink the whole bottle!

But let's return to your meals. They should be your primary source of sirtuin-activating nutrients, so they have an essential part of this diet. Unlike fasting, the sirtfood food doesn't force you to skip any meal, at least not in the maintenance phase. You can have all three meals during the day, but make sure you have the meals at regular times. This means that if you are having lunch at 1:00 p.m. on Monday, you shouldn't have lunch at 3:00 p.m. on Tuesday. Try to stick to the meal schedule, even though you have a hectic work schedule. When you are having just one green juice per day, the best time to have it is only 30 minutes before your breakfast. This is to maximize the absorption of sirtuin-activating nutrients. Others may prefer to have this juice between breakfast and lunch, but in this case, you need to wait two or three hours after your breakfast. Anyway, the sirtfood diet is all about flexibility, so it allows you to choose the time when to have the green juice.

But there are other ways to increase the sirtuin-activating nutrients intake. You can simply have some Sirt food bites or snacks. You can have meals more frequently (in smaller quantities), or you can have one or two more substantial snacks per day. But now you may be probably wondering what these Sirt food bites or snacks are. You can easily include in this category meals made of walnuts, cocoa, turmeric, dates, and extra-virgin olive oil. The general recommendation is to have one to two meals (more consistent) per day.

The food you can eat is not limited to the recipes you can find. You can easily improvise and "sirtify" your food. There are a few tricks to increase the sirtuin-activating nutrients from your diet. You can easily add sirtfoods on the plate to boost the health benefits of the meal. Think of simple breakfast pancakes. A way to "Sirtify" it is to add dark chocolate sauce or put some strawberries or walnuts on top. On a regular pizza, you can add a proper garlic sauce or capers. When it comes to drinks, a good trick is to create a refreshing drink by adding strawberries to sparkling or still water. You may add an extra coffee per day if you wish, but the real catch when it comes to Sirt food drinks is to abuse matcha green tea.

Cooking for yourself is somewhat tricky, as you have to be careful when splitting the quantities. Buy less and more frequently. The easiest way to stick to the Sirt food diet is to have somebody "sharing the burden" with you. If you can convince your partner to stick to the same menu, everything is more straightforward for you, as you will cook for more people, and you will have a higher motivation to stick to your diet. It would even be better if you can prepare for more people. So far, no studies are showing that the Sirt food diet should not be tried by a growing body (children, teenagers, pregnant, or breastfeeding women).

Since you have a hectic lifestyle, cooking can be done mostly in the evenings. Therefore, make sure you cook efficiently for more people and more servings. Share the health and weight-loss benefits of this diet with other people from your family.

Breakfast

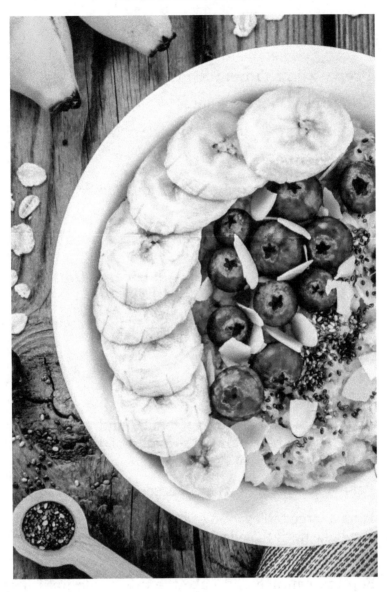

Vanilla Protein Pancakes

Preparation Time: 20 minutes

Cooking Time: 15 minutes

Servings: 8

Ingredients:

1½ cups Pea protein isolate

½ cup Whole wheat flour

1½ cups Almond milk (can be substituted with water)

2 tsp. Baking powder

2 tsp. Vanilla extract

Optional Toppings:

Walnuts

Blueberries (fresh or frozen)

Shredded coconut

Directions:

Add all ingredients to a blender and blend until smooth, scraping down the sides of the mixer to prevent any lumps if necessary.

Put a non-stick frying pan over medium heat.

Pour a large tablespoon of batter into the frying pan and bake until the edges are dry and bubbles form in the pancake.

Flip the pancake and bake the other side until it's lightly browned.

Repeat the process for the remaining pancake batter.

Serve the pancakes with the optional toppings and enjoy!

Store the pancakes in a fridge and consume within three days. Alternatively, store in the freezer for an of 30 days and thaw at room temperature. Use a microwave or non-stick frying pan to reheat the pancakes before serving.

Nutrition: Calories: 120 Carbs: 9.0 g. Fat: 2.2 g. Protein: 18.2 g. Fiber: 2.4 g. Sugar: 1.2

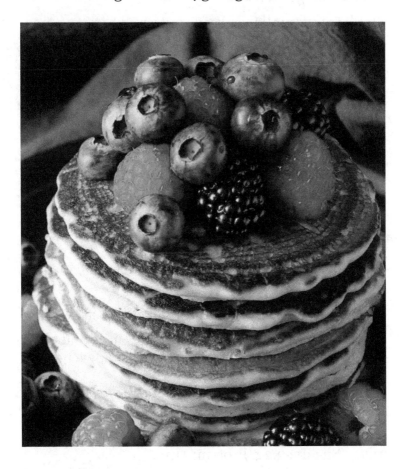

Morning Egg Sandwiches

Preparation Time: 10 minutes

Cooking Time: 10 minutes

Servings: 4

Ingredients:

5 oz. whole-grain bread

1 tablespoon sunflower seeds butter

¼ teaspoon salt

1 avocado, pitted

4 eggs

Directions:

Slice the bread into 8 slices.

Preheat a skillet and add the sunflower seeds butter and melt it well.

Beat the eggs in the skillet and sprinkle them with the salt.

Chop the avocado into the medium cubes and mash it well.

Spread the bread slices with the avocado mash.

When the eggs are cooked, cool them a little and place on top of the bread slices to make the sandwiches.

Serve the dish immediately.

Nutrition: Calories: 275, Fat: 17.7g, Total Carbs: 21.7g, Sugars: 3.2g, Protein: 11.1g

Quinoa Bowl

Preparation Time: 10 minutes

Cooking Time: 15 minutes

Servings: 6

Ingredients:

2 cups quinoa

1 cup blueberries

1 cup coconut milk, unsweetened

2 cups of water

2 tablespoons almonds

1 teaspoon pistachio

2 tablespoons honey

Directions:

Combine the coconut milk and water together in the saucepan and stir the liquid well.

Add the quinoa and close the lid.

Cook the mixture on medium heat for 5 minutes.

Wash the blueberries carefully and add them to the quinoa mixture.

Stir it carefully and continue to cook.

Combine the pistachio and almonds together and crush the nuts.

Sprinkle the quinoa with the crushed nuts and cook the mixture for 3 minutes more.

Add honey and stir the mixture carefully until the honey has dissolved.

Transfer to serving bowls and enjoy.

Nutrition: Calories: 348, Fat: 14.1g, Carbs: 48.3g, Sugars: 9.6g, Protein: 9.6g

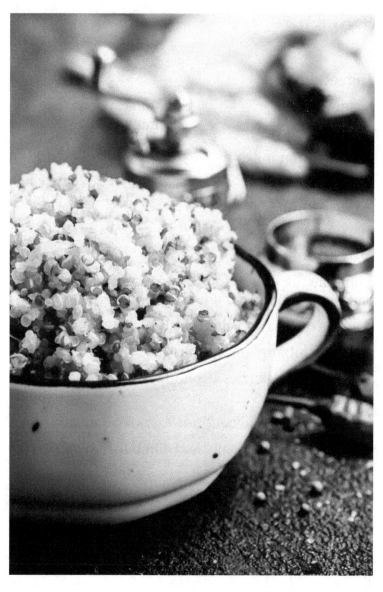

Sweet Potato Salad with Bacon

Preparation Time: 55 minutes
Cooking Time: 30 minutes
Servings: 1

Ingredients

5 slices Bacon

2 pieces Sweet potato (peeled and diced)

3 cloves Garlic (pressed)

4 tablespoon Lime juice

3 tablespoon Olive oil

1 tablespoon Balsamic vinegar

Directions:

Preheat the oven to 220 ° C and cover a baking sheet with parchment paper.

Place the bacon on the baking sheet and bake until crispy in the oven (approx. 20 minutes).

Take the bacon off the baking sheet, let it cool and chop it.

Mix the sweet potato cubes with garlic on the same baking sheet, drizzle with a little mild olive oil and fry them in the oven for about 30 minutes.

Prepare a dressing made from olive oil, vinegar, and lime juice by mixing them in a bowl.

Take the potato cubes out of the oven, mix them with the bacon pieces and drizzle them with the dressing.

If you like, add rocket and/or pine nuts at the end.

Nutrition: Calories: 205Total Fat: 5g Carbohydrate: 39g Protein: 4g

Turkey Breakfast Sausages

Preparation Time: 15 minutes
Cooking Time: 20 minutes
Servings: 2

Ingredients:

1 lb. extra lean ground turkey

1 Tbsp EVOO, and a little more to dirt pan

1 Tbsp fennel seeds

2 teaspoons smoked paprika

1 teaspoon red pepper flakes

1 teaspoon peppermint

1 teaspoon chicken seasoning

A couple of shredded cheddar cheese

A couple of chives, finely chopped

A few shakes garlic and onion powder

Two spins of pepper and salt

Directions:

Pre Heat oven to 350F.

Utilize a little EVOO to dirt a miniature muffin pan.

Combine all ingredients and blend thoroughly.

Fill each pit on top of the pan and then cook for approximately 15-20 minutes. Each toaster differs; therefore, when muffin fever is 165, then remove.

Nutrition: Calories: 168 Cal Fat: 44.71 g Protein: 285.92 g Sugar: 3.71 g

Peanut Butter, Banana Buckwheat Porridge

Preparation Time: 5 minutes
Cooking Time: 5 minutes
Servings: 1

Ingredients:

1/2 cup Buckwheat

1/2 cup milk, 2%

1/2 cup water

1 medium (7" to 7-7/8" long) Banana, fresh

1 tbsp Peanut Butter, smooth style, with salt

1 tbsp Coconut Flakes

Directions:

Soak buckwheat overnight the morning drain and rinse the buckwheat

Combine ingredient microwave for 1- 1.5 minutes

Nutrition: Calories: 190 Fat: 2.1g Fiber: 4g Carbs: 40g Protein: 4.1g

Green Omelet

Preparation Time: 5 minutes
Cooking Time: 5-10 minutes
Servings: 1

Ingredients:

1 tsp olive oil

1 shallot, peeled and finely chopped

2 large eggs, at room temperature

Handful (20g) rocket leaves

Small handful (10g) parsley, finely chopped

Salt and freshly ground black pepper

Directions:

In a wide frying pan: heat the oil on medium-low heat and gently fry the shallot for 5 minutes. Turn the heat up a little bit and cook for another 2 minutes.

In a bowl or cup, whisk the eggs together well with a fork. Distribute the shallot evenly around the pan before pouring m the eggs. Tip the pan slightly to each side so that the egg is evenly distributed. Cook for a minute or so before lifting the sides of the omelet and letting any runny egg slip into the base of the pan. Immediately sprinkle over the rocket leaves and parsley and season generously with salt and pepper. When cooked, the top of the omelet will still be soft but not runny, and the base will be just starting to brown. Tip onto a plate and enjoy straight away.

Nutrition: Calories: 220 Fat: 3.4g Fiber: 4,4g Carbs: 48.9g Protein: 6g

Sirt Muesli

Preparation Time: 5 minutes
Cooking Time: 0 minutes
Servings: 1

Ingredients:

1/4 cup buckwheat flakes

2/3 cup buckwheat puffs

3 tablespoons coconut flakes or dried coconut

1/4 cup Medjool dates, pitted and chopped

1/8 cup walnuts, chopped

1 ½ tablespoon cocoa nibs

2/3 cup strawberries, hulled and chopped

3/8 cup plain Greek yogurt (or vegan alternative,
such as soy or coconut yogurt)

Directions:

Mix all of the ingredients together (leave out the
strawberries and yogurt if not serving right away).

Nutrition: Calories: 176 Fat: 2.1g Fiber: 3.2g Carbs:
3.4g Protein: 5g

Sweet Oatmeal

Preparation Time: 5 minutes
Cooking Time: 10 minutes
Servings: 3

Ingredients:

1 cup oatmeal

5 apricots

1 tablespoon honey

1 cup coconut milk, unsweetened

1 teaspoon cashew butter

¼ teaspoon salt

½ cup of water

Directions:

Combine the coconut milk and oatmeal together in the saucepan and stir the mixture.

Add the water and stir it again. Sprinkle the mixture with the salt and close the lid.

Cook the oatmeal on medium heat for 10 minutes.

Meanwhile, chop the apricots into tiny pieces and combine the chopped fruit with the honey.

When the oatmeal is cooked, add cashew butter and fruit mixture.

Stir carefully and transfer to serving bowls.

Serve immediately.

Nutrition: Calories: 336, Fat: 21.2g, Total Carbs: 35.1g, Sugars: 14.0g, Protein: 6.2g

Green Beans and Eggs

Preparation Time: 10 minutes
Cooking Time: 15 minutes
Servings: 2

Ingredients:

½ cup green beans
¼ teaspoon salt
5 eggs
1/3 cup skim milk

1 bell pepper, seeds removed
1 teaspoon olive oil

Directions:

Slice the bell pepper and combine it with the green beans.

Pour the olive oil in a skillet and transfer the vegetable mixture to the skillet.

Cook on medium heat for 3 minutes, stirring frequently.

Meanwhile, beat the eggs in a mixing bowl.

Sprinkle the egg mixture with the salt and add skim milk. Whisk well.

Pour the egg mixture over the vegetable mixture and cook for 3 minutes on medium heat.

Stir the mixture carefully so that the eggs and vegetables are well combined.

Cook for 4 minutes more.

Stir again and close the lid.

Cook the scrambled eggs for 5 minutes more.

Stir the mixture again.

Serve it.

Nutrition: Calories: 231, Fat: 13.4g, Total Carbs: 9.3g, Sugars: 6.2g, Protein: 16.3g

Lunch

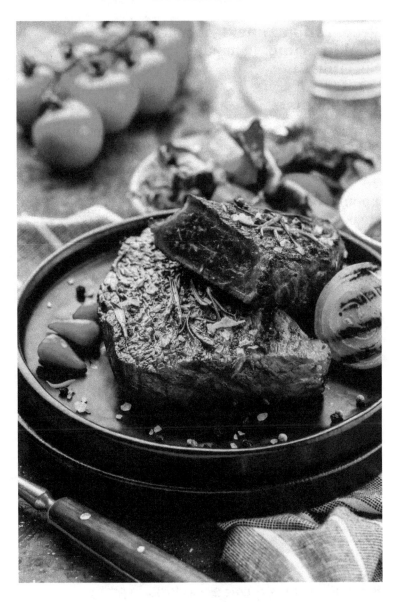

Steak with Veggies

Preparation Time: 15 minutes
Cooking Time: 12 minutes
Servings: 4

Ingredients:

2 tablespoons coconut oil

4 garlic cloves, minced

1 pound beef sirloin steak, cut into bite-sized pieces

Ground black pepper, as required

1½ cups carrots, peeled and cut into matchsticks

1½ cups fresh kale, tough ribs removed and chopped

3 tablespoons tamari

Directions:

Melt the coconut oil in a wok over medium heat and sauté the garlic for about 1 minute.

Add the beef and black pepper and stir to combine.

Increase the heat to medium-high and cook for about 3-4 minutes or until browned from all sides.

Add the carrot, kale and tamari and cook for about 4-5 minutes.

Remove from the heat and serve hot.

Nutrition: Calories 311 Total Fat 13.8 g Total Carbs 8.4 g Fiber 1.6 g Sugar 2.3 g Protein 37.1 g

Shrimps with Veggies

Preparation Time: 15 minutes
Cooking Time: 8 minutes
Servings: 5
Ingredients:

For Sauce:

1 tablespoon fresh ginger, grated

2 garlic cloves, minced

3 tablespoons low-sodium soy sauce

1 tablespoon red wine vinegar

1 teaspoon brown sugar

¼ teaspoon red pepper flakes, crushed

For Shrimp Mixture:

3 tablespoons olive oil

1½ pounds medium shrimp, peeled and deveined

12 ounces broccoli florets

8 ounces, carrot, peeled and sliced

Directions:

For sauce: in a bowl, place all the ingredients and beat until well combined. Set aside.

In a large wok, heat oil over medium-high heat and cook the shrimp for about 2 minutes, stirring occasionally.

Add the broccoli and carrot and cook about 3-4 minutes, stirring frequently.

Stir in the sauce mixture and cook for about 1-2 minutes.

Serve immediately.

Nutrition: Calories 298 Total Fat 10.7 g Total Carbs 7 g Protein 45.5 g

Kale apple and cranberry salad

Preparation Time: 15 minutes
Cooking Time: 0 minutes
Servings: 4

Ingredients

6 cups fresh baby kale

3 large apples, cored and sliced

¼ cup unsweetened dried cranberries

¼ cup almonds, sliced

2 tablespoons extra-virgin olive oil

1 tablespoon raw honey

Salt and ground black pepper, to taste

Directions:

In a salad bowl, place all the ingredients and toss to coat well.

Serve immediately.

Nutrition: Calories 253 Total Fat 10.3 g Total Carbs 40.7 g Fiber 6.6 g Sugar 22.7 g Protein 4.7 g

Arugula and Berries Salad

Preparation Time: 15 minutes
Cooking Time: 0 minutes
Servings: 4

Ingredients
1 cup fresh strawberries, hulled and sliced
½ cup fresh blueberries
½ cup fresh raspberries
6 cups fresh arugula
2 tablespoons extra-virgin olive oil
Salt and ground black pepper, to taste

Direction:
In a salad bowl, place all the ingredients and toss to coat well.
Serve immediately.

Nutrition: Calories 105 Total Fat 7.6 g Total Carbs 10.1 g Fiber 3.6 g Sugar 5.7 g Protein 1.6 g

Creamy Avocado and Chicken Spaghetti

Preparation Time: 15 minutes
Cooking Time: 15 minutes
Servings: 2

Ingredients:

12 oz spaghetti

1 cup cooked chicken, shredded

2 avocados, peeled and diced

1 cup cherry tomatoes, halved

1 garlic clove, chopped

2 tbsp basil pesto

5 tbsp olive oil

4 tbsp lemon juice

¼ cup grated parmesan cheese

Directions:

In a large pot of boiling salted water, cook spaghetti according to package directions. Drain and set aside in a large bowl.

In a blender, combine lemon juice, garlic, basil pesto, and avocados and blend until smooth.

Combine spaghetti, chicken, cherry tomatoes, and avocado sauce.

Sprinkle with parmesan cheese and serve immediately.

Nutrition: Calories: 285 Fat: 4.3g Fiber: 6g Carbs: 56g Protein: 8.5g

Chicken Breast in Tomato Salsa

Preparation Time: 10 minutes
Cooking Time: 15-20 minutes
Servings: 1

Ingredients:

1/4 pound skinless, boneless chicken bosom

2 teaspoons ground turmeric

juice of 1/4 lemon

1 tablespoon extra-virgin olive oil

3/4 cup kale, slashed

1/8 cup red onion, cut

1 teaspoon slashed new ginger

1/3 cup buckwheat

FOR THE SALSA

1 medium tomato

1 Thai beans, blanched

2 tablespoons parsley,

juice of 1/4 lemon

Directions:

Blend in with the stew, tricks, parsley, and lemon juice. You could place everything in a blender; however, the final product is somewhat extraordinary.

Marinate the chicken bosom in 1 teaspoon of the turmeric, the lemon juice, and a little oil. Leave for 5 to 10 minutes.

Warmth an ovenproof griddle until hot, at that point include the marinated chicken and cook for a moment or so on each side, until pale brilliant, at that point move to the broiler (place on a preparing plate if your dish isn't ovenproof) for 8 to 10 minutes or until cooked through.

Expel from the broiler, spread with foil, and leave to rest for 5 minutes before serving.

In the interim, cook the kale in a liner for 5 minutes. Fry the red onions and the ginger in a little oil, until delicate yet not seared, at that point include the cooked kale and fry for one more moment.

Cook the buckwheat as indicated by the bundle directions with the rest of the teaspoon of turmeric. Serve nearby the chicken, vegetables, and salsa.

Nutrition: Calories: 289 Fat: 3.5g Fiber: 5.3g Carbs: 45g Protein: 7g

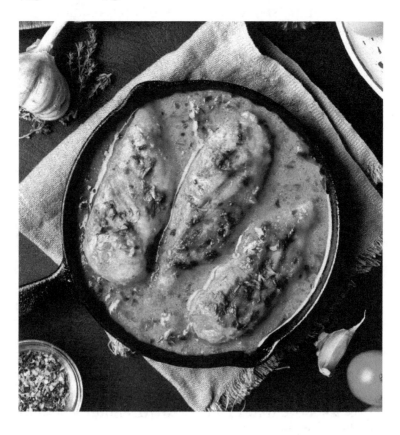

Tuscan Bean Stew

Preparation Time: 20 minutes
Cooking Time: 15 minutes
Servings: 2

Ingredients:

1 Chopped Italian Tomatoes

1.5 ounces Buckwheat

1 tablespoon Extra virgin olive oil

Vegetable stock - 200ml

Red onion - ¾ cup (finely chopped)

Carrot – ¼ cup (peeled and finely chopped)

Herbes de Provence - 1 teaspoon

Celery – 1 ounce (trimmed and finely chopped)

Garlic clove - 1 (finely chopped)

Tinned mixed beans – 1 cup

Bird's eye chilli - ½ (finely chopped), optional

Tomato purée - 1 teaspoon

Roughly chopped parsley - 1 tablespoon

Kale – ½ cup (roughly chopped)

Directions:

Pour the oil into a medium saucepan over low-medium heat. Once hot, add the onion, celery, carrot, herbs, garlic, and chilli and stir fry until the onion gets soft but not coloured.

Add the tomatoes, stock, and the tomato puree to the pan and bring to a boil. Add the beans and allow to simmer for thirty minutes.

Add the kale and cook for an additional 5 to 10 minutes, until tender. Now add the parsley.

In the casserole cook the buckwheat following the directions on the packet. Drain the water, then serve with the stew.

Nutrition: Calories: 250 Fat: 2g Fiber: 5.3g Carbs: 30g Protein: 12g

Sirtfood Cauliflower Couscous and Turkey Steak

Preparation Time: 45 minutes
Cooking Time: 10 minutes
Servings: 2

Ingredients:

5 ¼ oz cauliflower, roughly chopped

1 garlic clove, finely chopped

1 ½ oz. red onion, finely chopped

1 bird's eye chili, finely chopped

1 tsp. finely chopped fresh ginger

2 tbsp. extra virgin olive oil

2 tsp. ground turmeric

1 oz. sun dried tomatoes, finely chopped

⅜ oz parsley

5 ¼ oz. turkey steak

1 tsp. dried sage

Juice of ½ lemon

1 tbsp. capers

Directions:

Disintegrate the cauliflower using a food processor. Blend in 1-2 pulses until the cauliflower has a breadcrumb-like consistency.

In a skillet, fry garlic, chili, ginger and red onion in 1 tsp. olive oil for 2-3 minutes. Throw in the turmeric and cauliflower then cook for another 1-2 minutes.

Remove from heat and add the tomatoes and roughly half the parsley.

Garnish the turkey steak with sage and dress with oil. In a skillet, over medium heat, fry the turkey steak for 5 minutes, turning occasionally. Once the steak is cooked add lemon juice, capers and a dash of water. Stir and serve with the couscous.

Nutrition: Calories: 462 kcal Protein: 16.81 g Fat: 39.86 g Carbohydrates: 9.94 g

Chicken Thighs with Tomato Spinach Sauce

Preparation Time: 45 minutes
Cooking Time: 10 minutes
Servings: 2

Ingredients:

1 tablespoon olive oil

1.5 lb. chicken thighs, boneless skinless

½ teaspoon salt

¼ teaspoon pepper

8 oz. tomato sauce

Two garlic cloves, minced

½ cup overwhelming cream

4 oz. new spinach

Four leaves fresh basil (or utilize ¼ teaspoon dried basil)

Directions:

The most effective method to cook boneless skinless chicken thighs in a skillet: In a much skillet heat olive oil on medium warmth. Boneless chicken with salt and pepper. Add top side down to the hot skillet. Cook for 5 minutes on medium heat, until the high side, is pleasantly burned. Flip over to the opposite side and heat for five additional minutes on medium heat. Expel the chicken from the skillet to a plate. Step by step instructions to make creamy tomato basil sauce: To the equivalent, presently void skillet, include tomato sauce, minced garlic, and substantial cream. Bring to bubble and mix. Lessen warmth to low stew. Include new spinach and new basil. Mix until spinach withers and diminishes in volume. Taste the sauce and include progressively salt and pepper, if necessary. Include back cooked boneless skinless chicken thighs, increment warmth to medium.

Nutrition: Calories: 1061 kcal Protein: 66.42 g Fat: 77.08 g Carbohydrates: 29.51 g

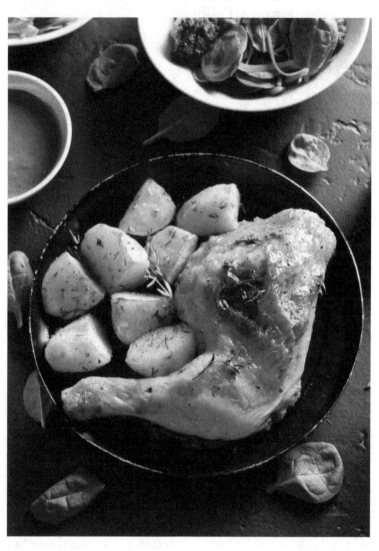

Chicken with Mole Salad

Preparation Time: 5 minutes
Cooking Time: 40 minutes
Servings: 2
Ingredients:

1 skinned chicken breast

2 cups spinach, washed, dried and torn in halves

2 celery stalks, chopped or sliced thinly

½ cup arugula

½ small red onion, diced

2 Medjool pitted dates, chopped

1 tbsp. of dark chocolate powder

1 tbsp. extra virgin olive oil

2 tbsp. water

5 sprigs of parsley, chopped

Dash of salt

Directions:

In a food processor, blend the dates, chocolate powder, oil and water, and salt. Add the chili and process further. Rub this paste onto the chicken breast, and set it aside, in the refrigerator.

Prepare other salad mixings, the vegetables and herbs in a bowl and toss.

Cook the chicken in a dash of oil in a pan, until done, about 10-15 minutes over a medium burner.

When done, let cool and lay over the salad bed and serve.

Nutrition: Calories 217 Total Fat 8.3 g Saturated Fat 1 g Cholesterol 0 mg

Dinner

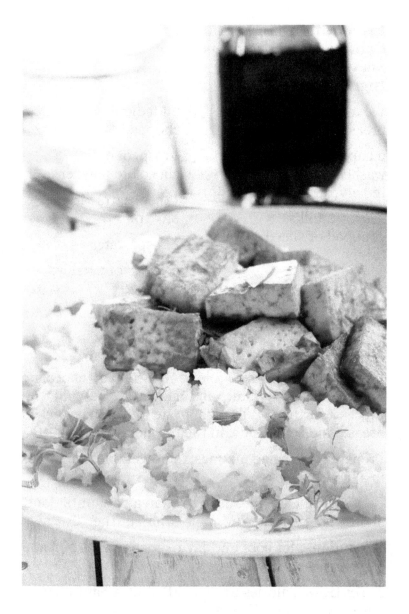

Tofu with Cauliflower

Preparation time: 5 minutes
Cooking time: 45 minutes
Servings: 2

Ingredients:

¼ cup red pepper, seeded
1 Thai chili, cut in two halves, seeded
2 cloves of garlic
1 tsp of olive oil
1 pinch of cumin
1 pinch of coriander
Juice of a half lemon
8oz tofu

8oz cauliflower, roughly chopped
1 ½oz red onions, finely chopped
1 tsp finely chopped ginger
2 teaspoons turmeric
1oz dried tomatoes, finely chopped
1oz parsley, chopped

Directions:

Preheat oven to 400 °F. Slice the peppers and put them in an ovenproof dish with chili and garlic.

Pour some olive oil over it, add the dried herbs and put it in the oven until the peppers are soft about 20 minutes).

Let it cool down, put the peppers together with the lemon juice in a blender and work it into a soft mass.

Cut the tofu in half and divide the halves into triangles.

Place the tofu in a small casserole dish, cover with the paprika mixture and place in the oven for about 20 minutes.

Chop the cauliflower until the pieces are smaller than a grain of rice.

Then, in a small saucepan, heat the garlic, onions, chili and ginger with olive oil until they become transparent. Add turmeric and cauliflower mix well and heat again.

Remove from heat and add parsley and tomatoes mix well. Serve with the tofu in the sauce.

Nutrition Facts: Calories 298kcal, Fat 5 g, Carbohydrate 55 g, Protein 27.5g

Sweet and Sour Pan

Preparation time: 30 minutes
Cooking time: 0 minutes
Servings: 2

Ingredients:

2 tbsp. Coconut oil

2 pieces Red onion

2 pieces yellow bell pepper

12oz White cabbage

6oz Pak choi

1 ½oz Mung bean sprouts

4 Pineapple slices

1 ½oz Cashew nuts

¼ cup Apple cider vinegar

4 tbsp. Coconut blossom sugar

1½ tbsp. Tomato paste

1 tsp Coconut-Aminos

2 tsp Arrowroot powder

¼ cup Water

Directions:

Roughly cut the vegetables. Mix the arrow root with five tbsp. of cold water into a paste.

Then put all the other ingredients for the sauce in a saucepan and add the arrowroot paste for binding.

Melt the coconut oil in a pan and fry the onion. Add the bell pepper, cabbage, pak choi and bean sprouts and stir-fry until the vegetables become a little softer.

Add the pineapple and cashew nuts and stir a few more times. Pour a little sauce over the wok dish and serve.

Nutrition Facts:

Calories: 573 kcal

Fat: 27.81 g

Carbohydrates: 77.91 g

Protein: 15.25 g

Vegetarian Curry

Preparation time: 15 minutes
Cooking time: 60 minutes
Servings: 2

Ingredients:

4 medium Carrots

2 medium Sweet potatoes

1 large Onion

3 cloves Garlic

4 tbsp. Curry powder

½ tsp caraway, ground

½ tsp Chili powder

Sea salt to taste

1 pinch Cinnamon

½ cup Vegetable broth

1 can Tomato cubes

8oz Sweet peas

2 tbsp. Tapioca flour

Directions:

Roughly chop carrots, sweet potatoes onions potatoes and garlic and put them all in a pot.

Mix tapioca flour with curry powder, cumin, chili powder, salt and cinnamon and sprinkle this mixture on the vegetables.

Add tomato cubes. Pour the vegetable broth over it.

Close the pot with a lid, bring to a boil and let it simmer for 60 minutes on a low heat. Stir in snap peas after 30min. Cauliflower rice is a great addition to this dish.

Nutrition Facts: Calories: 397 kcal Fat: 6.07 g Carbohydrates: 81.55 g Protein: 9.35 g

Goat's Cheese and Tomato Pizza

Preparation time: 5 minutes
Cooking time: 50 minutes
Servings: 2

Ingredients:

8oz buckwheat flour

2 teaspoons dried yeast

Pinch of salt

5fl oz. slightly water

1 teaspoon olive oil

For the Topping:

3 oz feta cheese, crumbled

3oz passata or tomato paste

1 tomato, sliced

1 red onion, finely chopped

1 oz rocket arugula leaves, chopped

Directions:

In a bowl, combine all the ingredients for the pizza dough then allow it to stand for at least an hour until it has doubled in size. Roll the dough out to a size to suit you. Spoon the passata onto the base and add the rest of the toppings. Bake in the oven at 200C/400F for 15-20 minutes or until browned at the edges and crispy and serve.

Nutrition: Calories: 269 kcal Protein: 9.23 g Fat: 23.76 g Carbohydrates: 5.49 g

Buckwheat with Onions

Preparation time: 10 minutes
Cooking time: 40 minutes
Servings: 4

Ingredients:

3 cups of buckwheat, rinsed

4 medium red onions, chopped

1 big white onion, chopped

5 oz. extra-virgin olive oil

3 cups of water

Salt and pepper, to taste

Direction:

Soak the buckwheat in the warm water for around 10 minutes. Then add in the buckwheat to your pot. Add in the water, salt and pepper to your pot and stir well.

Close the lid and cook for about 30-35 minutes until the buckwheat is ready. In the meantime, in a skillet, heat the extra-virgin olive oil and fry the chopped onions for 15 minutes until clear and caramelized.

Add some salt and pepper and mix well. Portion the buckwheat into four bowls or mugs. Then dollop each bowl with the onions. Remember that this dish should be served warm.

Nutrition Facts: Calories: 132; Fat: 32g;

Carbohydrates: 64g; Protein: 22g

Miso Caramelized Tofu

Preparation Time: 55 minutes
Cooking Time: 15 minutes
Servings: 2

Ingredients:

1 tbsp. mirin
3/4 oz. miso paste
5 1/4 oz. firm tofu
1 1/2 oz. celery, trimmed
1 1/4 oz. red onion
4 1/4 oz. zucchini
1 bird's eye chili
1 garlic clove, finely chopped

1 tsp. fresh ginger, finely chopped
1 5/8 oz. kale, chopped
2 tsp. sesame seeds
1 1/4 oz. buckwheat
1 tsp. ground turmeric
2 tsp. extra virgin olive oil
1 tsp. tamari (or soy sauce)

Directions

Pre-heat your over to 400°F. Cover a tray with parchment paper. Combine the mirin and miso together. Dice the tofu and let it marinate it in the mirin-miso mixture. Chop the vegetables (except for the kale) at a diagonal angle to produce long slices.

Using a steamer, cook for the kale for 5 minutes and set aside. Disperse the tofu across the lined tray and garnish with sesame seeds. Roast for 20 minutes, or until caramelized. Rinse the buckwheat using running water and a sieve.

Add to a pan of boiling water alongside turmeric and cook the buckwheat according to the packet instructions.

Heat the oil in a skillet over high heat. Toss in the vegetables, herbs and spices then fry for 2-3 minutes. Reduce to a medium heat and fry for a further 5 minutes or until cooked but still crunchy.

Nutrition Facts:

Calories: 101 kcal Fat: 4.7 g Carbohydrates: 12.38 g Protein: 4.22 g

Halibut with Garlic Spinach

Preparation Time: 10 minutes
Cooking Time: 7 minutes
Servings: 2

Ingredients:

2 (4-ounce) halibut fillets,

1 inch thick

½ lemon (about one teaspoon juice)

One teaspoon salt,

¼ teaspoon freshly ground black pepper (divided)

½ teaspoon cayenne pepper

1 teaspoon olive oil

2 cloves garlic

½ cup chopped red onion

2 cups fresh baby spinach leaves

Directions:

Preheat the broiler and place an oven rack 4 to 5 inches below the heat source. Line a baking sheet with aluminum foil.

Squeeze the lemon half over the fish fillets, then season each side with ½ teaspoon of the salt, pepper, and cayenne. Place the fish on the pan and broil for 7 to 8 minutes. Turn over the fish and cook for 6 to 7 minutes more, or until flaky.

Meanwhile, heat the olive oil in a small skillet over medium heat. Add the garlic and onion, and saute for 2 minutes. Add the spinach and remaining ½ teaspoon salt, and saute for 2 minutes more. Remove from the heat and cover to keep warm.

To serve, divide the spinach between two plates and top each portion with a fish fillet. Serve hot.

Nutrition: Fat 22g, Carbohydrates 17g, and Protein 19g

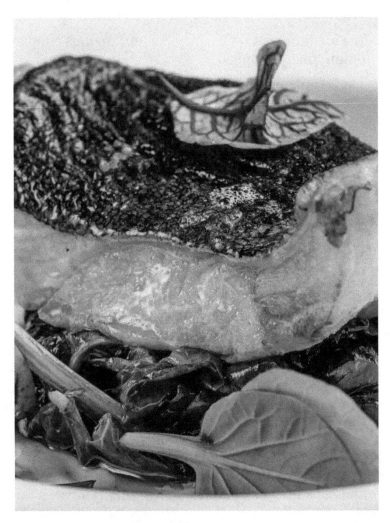

Quinoa Pilaf

Preparation Time: 30 minutes
Cooking Time: 20 minutes
Servings: 4

Ingredients

2 tablespoons extra virgin olive oil

1/2 medium yellow onion, finely chopped

1/4 bell pepper, finely chopped

1 garlic clove, minced

2 tablespoons pine nuts

1 cup uncooked quinoa

2 cups of water

Pinch freshly ground black pepper

2 tablespoons chopped fresh mint

2 tablespoons chopped fresh basil or Thai basil*

1 tablespoon chopped fresh chives (or green onions including the greens)

1 small cucumber, peeled, seeds removed, chopped

Salt and pepper

Directions:

Check your quinoa box, if you recommend washing it, place the quinoa in a large sieve and rinse it to remove water. (Some brands do not require washing). Onions, Peppers, garlic, pine nuts: Heat 1 tbsp. Put the olive oil over medium-high heat in a pot of 1/1 to 2 quarts. Add and cook onions, rusty peppers, garlic and pine nuts, occasionally stirring until the onions are translucent but not browned. Add quinoa: add and cook uncooked quinoa, occasionally stirring for a few minutes. You can toast a little quinoa for some bread. Add water, salt, stir: Add two glasses of water and a teaspoon of salt. Bring to a boil and reduce heat so that cheese and water shine while the pot is partially covered (enough for steam). Cook for 20 minutes or until quinoa is thin and liquid is absorbed. Remove from heat and serve in a large bowl. Fill with a fork. Add olive oil, mint, basil, onion, cucumber: add over low heat, add another tablespoon of olive oil. In chopped mint, mix basil, onion and cucumber. Add salt and pepper to taste. Chill or cool at room temperature.

Nutrition: Fat 22g, Carbohydrates 17g, and Protein 19g

Smoky Beans & Tempeh Patties

Preparation Time: 20 minutes
Cooking Time: 30 minutes
Servings: 4

Ingredients:

1 cup cooked cannellini beans
8 oz. tempeh
'¼ cup cooked bulgur
2 cloves garlic, pressed
¼ tsp onion powder
1 tsp liquid smoke
4 tsp Worcestershire sauce
1 tsp smoked paprika

2 tbsp. organic ketchup
2 tbsp. maple syrup
2 tbsp. neutral-flavored oil
3 tbsp. tamari.
¼ cup chickpea flour
Nonstick cooking spray

Directions:

Mash the beans in a large bowl: it's okay if a few small pieces of beans are left. Crumble the tempeh into small pieces on top. Add the bulgur and garlic.

In a medium bowl, whisk together the remaining ingredients, except the flour and cooking spray. Stir into the crumbled tempeh preparation. Add the flour and mix until well combined. Chill for 1 hour before shaping into patties.

Preheat the oven to 350°F. Line a baking tray with parchment paper. Scoop out 1/3 cup per patty, shaping into an approximately 3-inch circle and flattening slightly on the tray. You should get eight

3.5-inch patties in all. Lightly coat the top of the patties with cooking spray.

Bake for 15 minutes, carefully flip, and lightly coat the top of the patties with cooking spray and bake for another 15 minutes until lightly browned and firm.

Leftovers can be stored in an airtight container in the refrigerator for up to 4 days.

The patties can also be frozen, tightly wrapped in foil, for up to 3 months. If you don't eat all the patties at once, reheat the leftovers on low heat in a skillet lightly greased with olive oil or cooking spray for about 5 minutes on each side until heated through.

Nutrition Facts: Calories: 200kcal, Fat: 9g, Carbohydrate: 18g, Protein: 14g

Crispy Chickpeas with Green Beans

Preparation Time: 30 minutes
Cooking Time: 10 minutes
Servings: 4

Ingredients:

1 can chickpeas, rinsed

Kosher salt and freshly ground black pepper

1 tsp. whole coriander

1 tsp. cumin seeds

1 lb. green beans, trimmed

Grilled lemons, for serving

2 tbsp. olive oil, divided

Directions

Heat grill to medium. Gather chickpeas, coriander, cumin, and 1 tbsp. oil in a medium cast-iron skillet. Put skillet on grill and cook chickpeas, mixing occasionally, until golden brown and coriander begins to pop, 5 to 6 minutes. Season with salt and pepper.

Transfer to a bowl. Add green beans and remaining tbsp. olive oil to the skillet. Add salt and pepper. Cook, turning once, until charred and barely tender, 3 to 4 minutes.

Toss green beans with chickpea mixture and serve with grilled lemons alongside.

Nutrition: Calories: 460 Fat: 15g Carbs: 57g Protein: 16g

Dessert

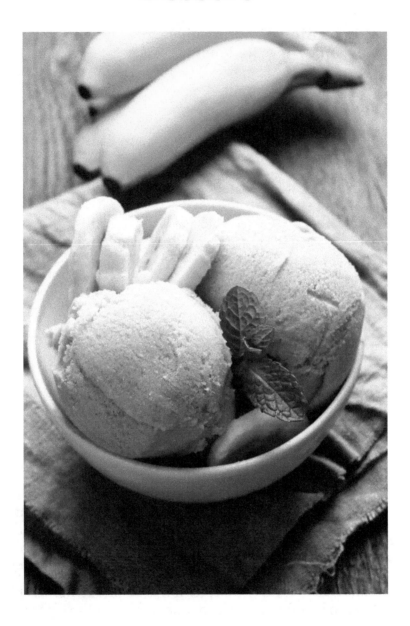

Lemon Ricotta Cookies

Preparation Time: 10 minutes
Cooking Time: 20 Minutes
Servings: 12

Ingredients:

2 1/2 cups all-purpose flour
1 tsp. baking powder
1 tsp. salt
1 tbsp. unsalted butter softened
2 cups of sugar
2 capsules
1 teaspoon (15-ounce) container whole-milk ricotta cheese
3 tbsp. lemon juice
1 lemon
Glaze:
11/2 cups powdered sugar
3 tbsp. lemon juice
1 lemon

Directions:

Pre heat the oven to 375 degrees f.

In a medium bowl combine the flour, baking powder, and salt. Set-aside.

From the big bowl blend the butter and the sugar levels. With an electric mixer beat the sugar and butter until light and fluffy, about three minutes. Add the eggs1 at a time, beating until incorporated.

Insert the ricotta cheese, lemon juice and lemon zest. Beat to blend. Stir in the dry skin.

Line two baking sheets with parchment paper. Spoon the dough (approximately 2 tablespoons of each cookie) on the baking sheets. Bake for fifteen minutes, until slightly golden at the borders. Remove from the oven and allow the biscuits remaining baking sheet for about 20 minutes.

Combine the powdered sugar lemon juice and lemon peel in a small bowl and then stir until smooth. Spoon approximately 1/2-tsp on each cookie and make use of the back of the spoon to lightly disperse. Allow glaze harden for approximately two hours. Pack the biscuits to a decorative jar.

Nutrition:
Carbs 24.5g
Protein 13.4g
Fat 2g

Banana Ice Cream

Preparation Time: 5 minutes
Cooking Time: 10 Minutes
Servings: 3 servings

Ingredients:

3 quite ripe banana - peeled and rooted

Couple of chocolate chips

Two tbsp. skim milk

Directions:

Throw all ingredients into a food processor and blend until creamy.

Eat freeze and appreciate afterwards.

Nutrition: Total fat 0.3g Carbs 23g Protein 3g

Matcha Mochi

Preparation Time: 1 minutes
Cooking Time: 20 Minutes
Servings: 2

Ingredients:

1 cup Superfine White Rice Flour

1 cup of coconut milk

2 tablespoons matcha powder

1/2 cup sugar

2 tablespoons butter melted

1 teaspoon baking powder

Directions:

Preheat the oven to 325.Spray baking dish with non-stick spray. (we use a coconut oil spray.). Mix all dry ingredients, including sugar. Whisk to blend. Add melted butter and coconut milk. Stir well. Put into a baking dish. We used an 8x8 pan. Bake for 20 minutes or until done in the middle.

Nutrition: Calories: 170Fat: 4,3g Fiber: 3.9g

Carbs: 34g Protein: 4.9g

Blueberry Muffins

Preparation Time: 15 minutes
Cooking Time: 25 Minutes
Servings: 10 servings

Ingredients:

1 cup Fresh blueberries

2 Tbsp Melted coconut oil

2 Tbsp Maple syrup

2 Eggs

5 cup Almond milk

A pinch of Salt

1.5 tsp Baking powder

¼ cup Arrowroot starch
1 cup Buckwheat flour

Directions:

Turn on the oven and let it heat up to 350 degrees. Prepare a muffin tin.

Bring out a bowl and add the salt, baking powder, arrowroot starch, and buckwheat flour.

Using a new bowl, mix the eggs, milk, oil, and syrup together. Beat them together until well combined. Add in the flour mixture and then fold in the blueberries.

Move to the muffin tins and then add into the oven. Bake for 25 minutes. When these are done, take them out to cool and then serve.

Brownie Bites

Preparation Time: 2 hours
Cooking Time: 0 Minutes
Servings: 12 pcs

Ingredients:

2½ cups whole walnuts

¼ cup almonds

2½ cups Medjoolodates

1 cup cacao powder

1 teaspoon vanilla extract

⅛-¼ teaspoon sea salt

Directions:

Place everything in a food processor until well combined.

Roll into balls and place on a baking sheet and freeze for 30 minutes or refrigerate for 2 hours.

Nutrition: Calories: 110 Fat: 2.8g Fiber: 4.1g

Carbs: 31.6g Protein: 5g

Mascarpone Cheesecake

Preparation Time: 10 minutes
Cooking Time: 20 Minutes
Servings: 3
Ingredients:

Crust
1/2 cup slivered almonds
8 tsp. -- or 2/3 cup graham cracker crumbs
2 tbsp. sugar
1 tbsp. salted butter melted
Filling
1 (8-ounce) packages cream cheese, room temperature
1 (8-ounce) container mascarpone cheese, room temperature
3/4 cup sugar
1 tsp. fresh lemon juice (or imitation lemon-juice)
1 tsp. vanilla infusion
2 large eggs, room temperature
Directions:

For the crust: preheat oven to 350 degrees f. Take per 9-inch diameter around the pan. Finely grind the almonds, cracker crumbs sugar in a food processor. Bring the butter and process until moist crumbs form.

Press the almond mixture on the base of the prepared pan (maybe not on the surfaces of the pan). Bake the crust until its put and start to brown, about 1-2 minutes. Cool. Decrease the oven temperature to 325 degrees f.

For your filling: with an electric mixer, beat the cream cheese, mascarpone cheese, and sugar in a large bowl until smooth, occasionally scraping down the sides of the jar using a rubber spatula. Beat in the lemon juice and vanilla. Add the eggs1 at a time, beating until combined after each addition.

Pour the cheese mixture on the crust from the pan. Put the pan into a big skillet or Pyrex dish pour enough hot water to the roasting pan to come halfway up the sides of one's skillet. Bake until the middle of this racket goes slightly when the pan is gently shaken, about 1 hour (the dessert will get business if it's cold). Transfer the cake to a stand; trendy for 1 hour. Refrigerate before cheesecake is cold, at least eight hours.

Topping squeezed just a small thick cream at the microwave using a busted-up chocolate brown -- afterward got a plastic bag and cut out a hole at the corner—then poured the melted chocolate to the baggie and used this to decorate the cake!

Nutrition: Calories: 250; Carbs 5g; Fat 25g; Protein 5g

Chocolate Berry Blend

Preparation Time: 30 Minutes
Cooking Time: 0 Minutes
Servings: 1

Ingredients:

2oz kale

2oz blueberries

2oz strawberries

1 banana

1 tablespoon 100% cocoa powder or cacao nibs

7 oz unsweetened soya milk

Directions:

Place all of the ingredients into a blender with enough water to cover them and process until smooth.

Nutrition: Calories: 256 Fats: 9g Carbs: 25g Proteins: 16g

Buckwheat Pancakes with Strawberries

Preparation Time: 25 Minutes
Cooking Time: 10 Minutes
Servings: 8

Ingredients:

1.5 cups soy milk
1 cup buckwheat flour
1 large egg
1 tablespoon extra-virgin olive oil, for cooking
1 ½ cups strawberries, chopped
For the chocolate nut butter:

2/3 cup dark chocolate (at least 85%)
¼ cup milk
2 tablespoons double cream
1 tablespoon coconut oil
½ cup walnuts

Directions:

Place milk, flour, and egg in a blender and blend until smooth. Transfer batter to measuring cup for easy pouring. To make the chocolate nut butter: melt chocolate in a double-boiler, once melted, whisk in the milk, then the double cream and oil. Pour into a blender with your walnuts and blend until smooth. For a saucier mix, add more milk or cream as desired. To make the pancakes: warm a griddle to medium heat, adding a small amount of oil as needed. Pour batter onto griddle and cook until lightly browned on the bottom. Watch for air bubbles. You will know it's time to flip your pancake when the air bubbles pop. Flip your pancakes and cook until lightly browned on the other side. Repeat with the remaining batter. Top pancakes with strawberries and drizzle over with sauce, as desired.

Nutrition: Calories: 278 Cal Fats: 15g Carbs: 15g Proteins: 24g

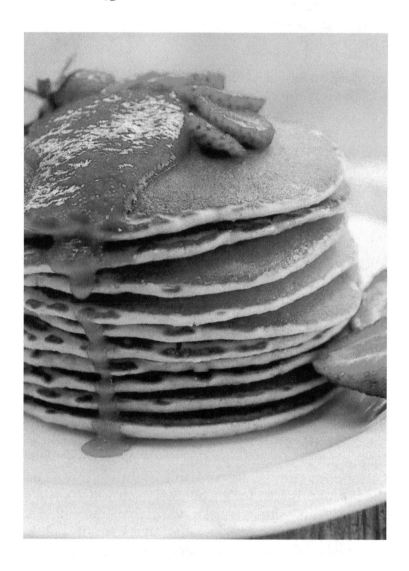

Apple Pancakes

Preparation Time: 20 Minutes
Cooking Time: 20 Minutes
Servings: 4

Ingredients:

Egg whites - 2

Plain flour – 1 cup

Porridge oats – ½ cup

Baking powder - 1 teaspoon

Pinch of salt

Sugar - 2 tablespoon

Apples – 2 (peeled, cored and chop into small pieces)

Light olive oil - 2 teaspoon

Semi-skimmed milk – 1 ½ cup

For the Compote

Blackcurrant– ½ cup (washed and stalks removed)

Water - 3 tablespoons

Sugar - 2 tablespoons

Directions:

The first step is to get your compote ready. Add the water, sugar, and blackcurrant into a small pan. Allow to simmer, and then cook for about 10 to 15 minutes. Add the baking powder, salt, caster sugar, flour, and oats in a large bowl. Mix thoroughly. Add the apples, stir, and then whisk in the milk, a little at a time until you have a smooth consistency. Whisk the egg whites to stiff peaks then add into the pancake batter. Move the batter into a jug. Heat half teaspoon of oil in a non-stick frying pan over medium-high heat. Begin by pouring in approximately one-quarter of the batter. Cook on both sides until the batter turns golden brown. Remove the set and add the next batch until you have four pancakes. Place the pancakes in a plate and drizzle the blackcurrant compote over them. Serve.

Nutrition: Calories: 337 Fats: 3g Carbs: 32g Proteins: 12g

Chocolate Coffee Mousse

Preparation Time: 2 hours
Cooking Time: 15 Minutes
Servings: 2

Ingredients:

4 oz dark chocolate (85% cocoa solids)

6 medium free-range eggs, separated

4 tbsp strong black coffee

4 tbsp almond milk

Chocolate coffee beans, to decorate

Directions:

Melt the chocolate in a large bowl set over a pan of gently simmering water, making sure the bottom of the bowl doesn't touch the water.

Remove the bowl from the heat and leave the melted chocolate to cool to room temperature. Once the melted chocolate is at room temperature, whisk in the egg yolks one at a time and then gently fold in the coffee and almond milk. Using a hand-held electric mixer, whisk the egg whites until stiff peaks form, then mix a couple of tablespoons into the chocolate mixture to loosen it. Gently fold in the remainder, using a large metal spoon. Transfer the mousse to individual glasses and smooth the surface. Cover with cling film and chill for at least 2 hours, ideally overnight. Decorate with chocolate coffee beans before serving.

Nutrition: Calories: 156 Fat: 3.1g Fiber: 3.9g

Carbs: 31g Protein: 3.6g

Snacks

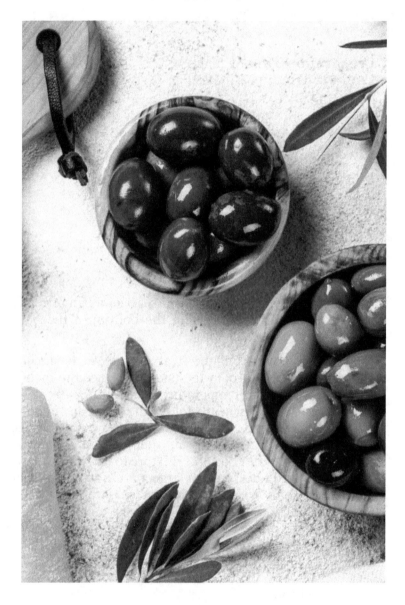

Med-Style Olives

Preparation Time: 10 minutes
Cooking Time: 10 minutes
Servings: 6

Ingredients:

One pinch of salt One pinch of black pepper

1 ½ tablespoon of coriander seeds

One tablespoon of extra-virgin olive oil

One lemon

7 oz. of kalamata olives

7 oz. of green queen olives

Directions:

Using a pestle and mortar, finely crush the coriander seeds and set aside.

Using a sharp knife, cut long, thin slices of lemon rind and place into a bowl with both the green queen and kalamata olives.

Squeeze the juice of one lemon over the top of the olives and add the olive oil.

Add the salt, pepper, and coriander seeds, then stir and serve.

The longer you allow the olives to rest in the marinade, the more delicious they will taste.

Nutrition: Calories: 477;Total Fat: 9g;
Carbohydrate: 60g; Dietary Fiber: 3g; Protein: 35g

Roasted Chickpeas

Preparation Time: 10 minutes
Cooking Time: 40 minutes
Servings: 6
Ingredients:

One pinch of salt

One pinch of black pepper

One pinch of garlic powder

One teaspoon of dried oregano

Two tablespoons of extra-virgin olive oil

juice of 1 lemon

Two teaspoons of red wine vinegar

2 15 oz. canned chickpeas

Directions:

Preheat your oven to 42 5°F and place a sheet of parchment paper onto a baking tray.

Drain and rinse the chickpeas, then pour them onto the baking tray. Spread them evenly. Place them in the oven and roast them for 10 minutes. Remove from the oven, give the plate a firm shake, then return the plate to the oven for a further 10 minutes. Once roasted, remove from the oven and set aside. Add the remaining ingredients into a mixing bowl. Combine well, then add the roasted chickpeas. Using a spatula ensures that the chickpeas are evenly coated. Return the chickpeas into the oven and allow to roast for 10 minutes. Remove them from the oven, allow to cool, then serve.

Keep checking on the chickpeas while they roast to ensure they do not burn or require longer cooking time.

Nutrition: Calories: 323; Total fat: 15.6g; Carbohydrate: 39.5g; Protein: 10.4g

Honey Chili Nuts

Preparation Time: 10 minutes
Cooking Time: 30 minutes
Servings: 4

Ingredients:

5oz walnuts

5oz pecan nuts

2oz softened butter

1 tablespoon honey

½ bird's-eye chili, very finely chopped and deseeded

Directions:

Preheat the oven to 180C/360F. Combine the butter, honey, and chili in a bowl, then add the nuts and stir them well. Spread the nuts onto a lined baking sheet and roast them in the oven for 10 minutes, stirring once halfway through. Remove from the oven and allow them to cool before eating.

Nutrition: Calories: 65g Fat: 0.5g Fiber: 0.8g Carbs: 4.9g Protein: 2g

Cauliflower Nachos

Preparation Time: 5 minutes
Cooking Time: 30 minutes
Servings: 1-2

Ingredients:

2 tablespoons extra virgin olive oil

½ teaspoon onion powder

½ teaspoon turmeric

½ teaspoon ground cumin

1 medium head cauliflower

¾ cup shredded cheddar cheese

½ cup tomato, diced

¼ cup red bell pepper, diced

¼ cup red onion, diced

½ Bird's Eye chili pepper, finely diced

¼ cup parsley, finely diced

Pinch of salt

Directions:

Preheat oven to 400 ° F.

Mix onion powder, cumin, turmeric, and olive oil. Core cauliflower and slice into ½" thick rounds. Coat the cauliflower with the olive oil mixture and bake for 15 – 20 minutes. Top with shredded cheese & bake for an additional 3 – 5 minutes, until cheese is melted. In a bowl, combine tomatoes, bell pepper, onion, chili, and parsley with a pinch of salt.

Top cooked cauliflower with salsa and serve.

Nutrition: Calories: 195g Fat: 5.1g Fiber: 5.3 Carbs: 50.9g Protein: 3.6g

Mozzarella Cauliflower Bars

Preparation Time: 10 minutes
Cooking Time: 40 minutes
Servings: 1

Ingredients:

½ cauliflower head, riced

1/3 cup low-fat mozzarella cheese, shredded

¼ cup egg whites

1 teaspoon Italian dressing, low fat

Pepper to taste

Directions:

Spread cauliflower rice over a lined baking sheet. Preheat your oven to 375 degrees F. Roast for 20 minutes. Transfer to a bowl and spread pepper, cheese, seasoning, egg whites, and stir well. Spread in a rectangular pan and press. Transfer to oven and cook for 20 minutes more. Serve and enjoy!

Nutrition: Calories: 90 Fat: 4g Fiber: 1.7g Carbs: 3.8g Protein: 4g

Walnut and Date Bites

Preparation Time: 5 minutes
Cooking Time: 0 minutes
Servings: 1

Ingredients:

3 walnut halves

3 pitted Medjool dates

the ground cinnamon, to taste

Directions:

Cut each walnut carefully into three slices, and do the same with dates. Put a slice of walnut, brush with cinnamon, and serve.

Nutrition: Calories: 78g Fat: 7g Fiber: 0,9g

Carbs: 3.4g Protein: 1.5g

Sirt Energy Balls

Preparation Time: 5 minutes
Cooking Time: 5 minutes
Servings: 2-4

Ingredients:

1 cup old fashion ginger, dried

1/4 cup quinoa cooked using 3/4 cup orange juice

1/4 cup shredded unsweetened coconut

1/3 cup dried cranberry/raisin blend

1/3 cup dark chocolate chips

1/4 cup slivered almonds

1 Tbsp reduced-fat peanut butter

Directions:

Cook quinoa in orange juice. Bring to boil and simmer for approximately 1-2 minutes. Let cool. Combine chilled quinoa and the remaining ingredients into a bowl.

With wet hands and combine ingredients and roll in golden ball sized chunks.

Set at a Tupperware and set in the refrigerator for two weeks until the firm.

Nutrition: Calories: 80 Fat: 7g Fiber: 1g Carbs: 3,5g

Protein: 2.5g

Celery and Raisins Snack Salad

Preparation Time: 10 minutes
Cooking Time: 0 minutes
Servings: 4

Ingredients:

½ cup raisins

4 cups celery, sliced

¼ cup parsley, chopped

½ cup walnuts, chopped

Juice of ½ lemon

2 tbsp. extra virgin olive oil

Salt and black pepper to the taste

Directions:

In a salad bowl, mix celery with raisins, walnuts, parsley, lemon juice, oil, and black pepper, toss, divide into small cups and serve as a snack.

Nutrition Facts: Calories 120 Fat 1g

Carbohydrate 6 g Protein 5 g

Smoothies

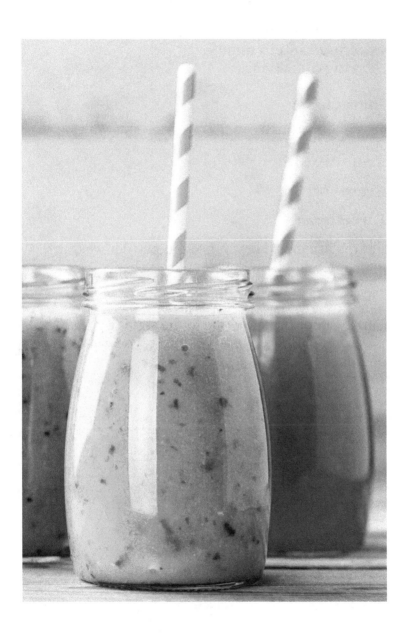

Berry Smoothie

Preparation Time: 5 minutes
Cooking Time: 1 minute
Servings: 1 Servings

Ingredients:

Two scoops Protein Powder 2 cups Almond Milk

4 cups Mixed Berry

2 cups Yoghurt

Directions:

First, place mixed berry, protein powder, yoghurt, and almond milk in the blender pitcher.

Then, select the 'smoothie' button.

Finally, pour the smoothie to the serving glass. To make it more nutritious and filling, you can even add banana to it.

Nutrition: Calories: 306 Carbs: 36g Fat: 3g Protein: 36g

Tofu Smoothie

Preparation Time: 5 minutes
Cooking Time: 5 Minutes
Servings: 2 Servings

Ingredients:

1 Banana, sliced & frozen

3/4 cup Almond Milk

2 tbsp. Peanut Butter

1/2 cup Yoghurt, plain & low-fat

1/2 cup Tofu, soft & silken

1/3 cup Dates, chopped

Directions:

First, place tofu, banana, dates, yogurt, peanut butter, and almond milk in the blender pitcher.

After that, press the 'smoothie' button.

Finally, transfer to serving glass and enjoy it.

Tip: You can try adding herbs to your preference.

Nutrition: Calories: 119 Sugar: 13 g.Fat: 2 g. Carbohydrates: 22 g. Fiber: 3 g. Protein: 5 g.

Grape Smoothie

Preparation Time: 5 minutes
Cooking Time: 0 minutes
Servings: 1

Ingredients:

2 cups red seedless grapes

¼ cup fruit juice

½ cup plain yogurt

1 cup ice

Directions:

Add fruit juice to the blender. At that time, put in the yogurt and grapes. Add the ice last. Blend until smooth, and enjoy!

Nutrition:

Calories: 160

Fat: 4.1g

Fiber: 1.5g

Carbs: 40g

Protein: 2.5

Black Forest Smoothie

Preparation Time: 5 minutes
Cooking Time: 0 minutes
Servings: 1

Ingredients:

50 g or ¼ cup frozen cherries

1 handful kale

1 Medjool date

2 tsp cocoa powder

1 tsp chia seeds

120 ml or ½ cup milk or soya milk

Directions:
Place all the ingredients into a blender and process until smooth and creamy.

Nutrition: Calories: 145g Fat: 2.5g

Fiber: 3g Carbs: 57.9g Protein: 1g

Celery Smoothie

Preparation Time: 5 minutes
Cooking Time: 0 minutes
Servings: 1

Ingredients:

2 stalks celery

2 cups cabbage

2 tbsp lemon juice

1 tsp dried dill

½ tsp juniper berries

Extra Water – optionally added to dilute the consistency

Directions:

Place all ingredients together in a blender and blend thoroughly. Serve chilled and enjoy!

Nutrition: Calories: 125.1g Fat: 1.2g

Fiber: 4.3g Carbs: 38g Protein: 3.1g

Kale and Cucumber Smoothie

Preparation Time: 5 minutes
Cooking Time: 0 minutes
Servings: 1

Ingredients:

1 handful kale

2-inch cucumber – sliced, chopped

Half-squeezed lime

1 medium mango, peeled & chopped

1 tablespoon goji berries

Extra Water – optionally added to dilute the consistency

Directions:

Place all ingredients together in a blender and blend thoroughly. Serve chilled and enjoy!

Nutrition: Calories: 125 Fat: 1.4g Fiber: 6g

Carbs: 34g Protein: 7g

Carrot Strawberry Smoothie

Preparation Time: 5 minutes
Cooking Time: 5 Minutes
Servings: 2

Ingredients:

1/3 cup Bell Pepper, diced

1 cup Carrot Juice, chilled

1 cup Mango, diced

1 cup Strawberries, unsweetened & frozen

Directions:

To start with, place strawberries, bell pepper, and mango in the blender pitcher.

After that, pulse it a few times.

Next, pour the carrot juice into it.

Finally, press the 'smoothie' button.

Tip: You can try adding pineapple chunks to it for enhanced flavor.

Nutrition: Calories: 70 Carbs: 25 g Fat: 1 g

Protein: 10 g

Green Smoothie

Preparation time: 5 minutes
Cooking time: 5 minutes
Servings: 3 to 4

Ingredients:

1/4 cup Baby Spinach

1/2 cup Ice

1/4 cup Kale

1/2 cup Pineapple Chunks

1/2 cup Coconut Water

1/2 cup mango, diced

1/2 Banana, diced

Directions:

Begin by placing all the ingredients needed to make the smoothie in the blender pitcher.

Now, press the 'extract' button.

Transfer the smoothie into the serving glass.

Nutrition: Calories: 207 Carbs: 33 g Fat: 2 g

Protein: 15 g Sugar: 25 g

Yogurt & Fruit Jam Parfait

Preparation time: 5 minutes
Cooking time: 5 minutes
Servings: 6

Ingredients:

3 cups Mixed Berries

1 tbsp. Lemon Juice

7/8 cup Honey

2 tsp. Fruit Pectin

1 cup Granola

3 cups Greek Yoghurt

Directions:

For making this healthy jam, you need to place the mixed berries, honey, lemon juice, and pectin in the blender pitcher.

Next, pulse the mixture 3 to 4 times and then press the 'sauce/ dip' button.

Now, transfer the jam to a safe heat container and then place it in the refrigerator for 2 to 3 hours.

Once the jam is chilled, layer 1/3 cup of the Greek Yoghurt into the bottom of the parfait glass.

After that, spoon in a jam into it and then add the granola.

Serve immediately.

Tip: If you don't want to use honey, you can use 1 cup of granulated sugar.

Nutrition: 154 calories; Carbs: 33 g Fat: 2 g Proteins 20g

Kiwi Smoothie

Preparation time: 5 minutes
Cooking time: 5 minutes
Servings: 3

Ingredients:

1/4 of 1 Avocado, ripe & pitted

1/4 cup Ice

1/4 cup Coconut Water

3/4 cup Kale Leaves

1/2 cm Ginger, fresh & peeled

2 Kiwis, quartered

1 Date pitted & halved

1 tsp. Lime Juice

Directions:

First, place ice, kale leaves, avocado, dates, kiwis, lime juice, ginger, and coconut water in the blender pitcher.

Then, press the 'smoothie' button.

Finally, transfer to a serving glass and enjoy it.

Nutrition: Calories: 268.0 Total Fat: 2.3 gTotal Carbs: 34.3 g Dietary Fiber: 6.0 g Protein: 27.9 g

Antioxidant Smoothie

Preparation Time: 5 minutes
Cooking Time: 5 minutes
Servings: 3

Ingredients:

1/2 cup Celery Stalk, halved

1/3 cup Watermelon, chopped into chunks

1/4 cup Ice

1/8 cup Red Cabbage, chopped

1/2 cup Blueberries

1/2 cup Pomegranate Juice

1/2 of 1 Apple, unpeeled & halved

Directions:

Begin by placing ice, red cabbage, celery stalk, apple, blueberries, and watermelon in the blender pitcher.

Now, select the 'smoothie' button.

Finally, transfer the smoothie to the serving glass and enjoy it.

Nutrition: Calories: 225.3 Total Fat: 9.1 g

Cholesterol: 10.0 mg Total Carbs: 29.7 g

Dietary Fiber: 7.2 g Protein: 9.1 g

4 Weeks Meal Plan

This is without any doubt the most important section of the Book, where you will be able to learn about your new healthy way of eating in the next 4 weeks.

Here you will fully understand what following a Sirtfood Diet means and find out how easy it is to reach your goals while making significant and lifetime changes that will guarantee weight loss results that last and an improved health condition.

Just follow the instructions and the month will fly by without even noticing it.

But before starting, let's talk about pantry basics.

Pantry Basics

The following ingredients are probably already in your pantry.

If not, add them <u>once</u> to have them handy during the next 4 weeks (but most of them will last much longer, even months).

Cooking basics:

Baking powder, Basmati rice Bread Crumbs, Brown Rice, Capers, Cocoa powder, Canned Tomatoes, Coconut Oil, Cooking Spray, Extra Virgin Olive Oil,

Flour, Honey, Oats, Red wine, Sesame oil, Stock cubes, Tomato sauce.

Dressings:

Balsamic Vinegar, Mustard, Salt, Soy Sauce, Tamari.

Herbs and Spices:

Bay, Basil, Chili, Cinnamon, Cumin, Curry, Dill, Garam Masala, Garlic, Ginger, Marjoram, Nutmeg, Oregano, Paprika, Pepper, Rosemary, Sage, Thyme, Turmeric, Vanilla Extract.

Nuts and Seeds:

Almonds, Pumpkin seeds, Sesame seeds, Walnuts.

Week one – Phase 1

This week is divided in two moments:

Day 1-3 with 3 juices a day, 1 optional snack and a full meal.

Day 4-7 with 2 juices a day, 2 optional snacks and a full meal.

Shopping List

Important: The Plan lets you choose your favorite Sirtfood Green Juices Recipes each week, remember to include the related ingredients in this list accordingly.

Artichokes	Chicken Thighs
Arugula	Chicken Wings
Avocado	Chicory
Baby Spinach	Coconut cream
Bird's eye chili	Dates
Broccoli	Goat Cheese
Buckwheat	Kale
Buckwheat flour	Lettuce
Carrots	Leeks
Celeriac	Lemons
Celery	Orange
Chicken Breast	Parmesan

Parsley

Red Onions

Red Peppers

Salmon

Shrimps

Smoked Salmon

Spinach

Sweet potatoes

Tomatoes

Tuna Steak

Turkey Breast

Turnips

Yellow Peppers

Week 2-3 Phase 2

This week is divided in two moments:

Week 2 with 1 juice a day, 2 optional snacks and 2 full meals.

Week 3 with 1 juice a day, 2 optional snacks and 2 full meals.

Shopping List

Important: The Plan lets you choose your favorite Sirtfood Green Juices Recipes each week, remember to include the related ingredients in this list accordingly.

Almond Milk, unsweetened	Carrots
Arugula	Cauliflower
Asparagus	Celeriac
Avocado	Celery
Baby Spinach	Cherry tomatoes
Banana	Chicken Wings
Bird's eye chili	Chicory
Blueberries	Chocolate, 85%
Broccoli	Coconut milk, full fat
Buckwheat, puffed	Cucumber
	Eggs

Greek yoghurt

Kale

Lean Mince

Lettuce

Lemons

Lentils, canned

Lime

Milk, skimmed

Mixed Berries, frozen

Mozzarella

Mushrooms

Oats

Orange

Parmesan

Parsley

Parsnip

Red Onions

Red Peppers

Salmon fillets

Scallions

Shrimps

Sirloin

Strawberries

Tomatoes

Trout fillets

Turkey Breast

Turnips

Yellow Peppers

Week 4 - Phase 3

After completing successfully Phase 1 and 2, Phase 3 will allow you to transition to normal healthy eating that keep including a variety of Sirtfoods in daily meals.

Week 4: 1 juice a day, 2 snacks and 3 full meals.

Shopping List

<u>Important:</u> The Plan lets you choose your favorite Sirtfood Green Juices Recipes each week, remember to include the related ingredients in this list accordingly.

Almond Milk, unsweetened

Almond Flour

Arugula

Avocado	Cheddar
Baby potatoes	Chicken Breast
Baby Spinach	Chicken Mince
Banana	Chickpeas, canned
Blueberries	Chicory
Broccoli	Coconut, shredded
Brussels Sprouts	Dates
Buns, whole wheat	Eggs
Butternut Squash	Lamb, shoulder
Buckwheat	Lean Mince

Lettuce

Lentils, canned

Mozzarella

Mushrooms

Oats

Parmesan

Parsley

Peanut Butter

Potatoes

Red Onions

Red Peppers

Ricotta cheese

Shrimps

Spinach

Strawberries

Sweet potatoes

Tomatoes

Tuna Steak

Wine

Conclusion

Congratulations, all stages of the Sirtfood Diet have now finished!

Just let's take a look of what you have achieved. You've entered the hyper-success phase 1, probably achieving a remarkable weight loss around 7 pounds and an interesting increase of muscle mass.

You also maintained your weight loss throughout the fourteen-day maintenance phase 2 and further improved your body composition. You have marked the beginning of your lifetime transformation thanks to phase 3, where you had a sample of how your new way of eating could be.

You took a stand against diseases which strikes often as we get older, enhancing your strength, productivity, and health.

By now, you are familiar with the top twenty Sirtfoods, and you've gained a sense of how powerful they are. Not only that, you probably have become quite good at including them in your diet and loving them. For the sustained weight loss and health, they offer, these items must stay a prominent feature in your everyday eating regimen.

Good luck to you as you move towards the new chapter of your healthy, happy life!